*Acting Edition*

# The Good Life

## by Mike Birbiglia

**FOR PRODUCTION INQUIRIES**

UNITED STATES AND CANADA
info@concordtheatricals.com
1-866-979-0447

UNITED KINGDOM AND EUROPE
licensing@concordtheatricals.co.uk
020-7054-7298

Each title is subject to availability from Concord Theatricals Corp., depending upon country of performance. Please be aware that *THE GOOD LIFE* may not be licensed by Concord Theatricals Corp. in your territory. Professional and amateur producers should contact the nearest Concord Theatricals Corp. office or licensing partner to verify availability.

No one shall make any changes in this title(s) for the purpose of production. No part of this book may be reproduced, stored in a retrieval system, scanned, uploaded, or transmitted in any form, by any means, now known or yet to be invented, including mechanical, electronic, digital, photocopying, recording, videotaping, or otherwise, without the prior written permission of the publisher. No one shall share this title(s), or any part of this title(s), through any social media or file hosting websites.

For all inquiries regarding motion picture, television, online/digital and other media rights, please contact Concord Theatricals Corp.

### MUSIC AND THIRD-PARTY MATERIALS USE NOTE

Licensees are solely responsible for obtaining formal written permission from copyright owners to use copyrighted music and/or other copyrighted third-party materials (e.g. artworks, logos) in the performance of this play and are strongly cautioned to do so. If no such permission is obtained by the licensee, then the licensee must use only original music and materials that the licensee owns and controls. Licensees are solely responsible and liable for clearances of all third-party copyrighted materials, including without limitation music, and shall indemnify the copyright owners of the play(s) and their licensing agent, Concord Theatricals Corp., against any costs, expenses, losses and liabilities arising from the use of such copyrighted third-party materials by licensees. For music, please contact the appropriate music licensing authority in your territory for the rights to any incidental music.

### IMPORTANT BILLING AND CREDIT REQUIREMENTS

If you have obtained performance rights to this title, please refer to your licensing agreement for important billing and credit requirements.

*THE GOOD LIFE* was first performed at the Beacon Theatre in New York City on March 22, 2025. It was written and performed by Mike Birbiglia. The executive producers were Joseph Birbiglia and John Skidmore; the consulting producer was J. Hope Stein; co-producers were Mabel Lewis, Peter Salomone, and Gary Simons. The performance was directed by Seth Barrish, with production design by Beowulf Boritt, lighting design by Aaron Copp, and a backdrop painted by Irina Portnyagina. Ira Glass served as story consultant.

Special thanks to Pope Francis (1936–2025)

# CHARACTER

**MIKE**


## AUTHOR'S NOTE

I've written six solo plays over the last twenty years. *Sleepwalk With Me, My Girlfriend's Boyfriend, Thank God For Jokes, The New One, The Old Man and the Pool,* and *The Good Life.* These shows were all directed by Seth Barrish and staged in New York City – on and off-Broadway – and all over the world. The aesthetic that Seth and I developed through the years is deliberate, and at its best, invisible. In other words, the direction isn't often seen but ideally is felt. At different points in the process, we considered incorporating larger set elements, but in the end, we always tried to stage the shows simply. This was done with the help of our brilliant designers Beowulf Boritt, Aaron Copp, and others. However, the way we staged the show is just one approach. Seth and I would love to see a production like that or a production that is very different from that. We would love to see productions starring any number of actors and any type of actor (regardless of race, gender, etc.). The goal for these solo shows is to attempt to have a connection in the room with the audience. However you can make that happen, we are excited to see it.


## NOTE ON TEXT

Text in [square brackets] is from the original production of *The Good Life* and is customized to the specifics of the Broadway venue and city where it was performed. Take liberties in customizing these moments to your specific theater and city.

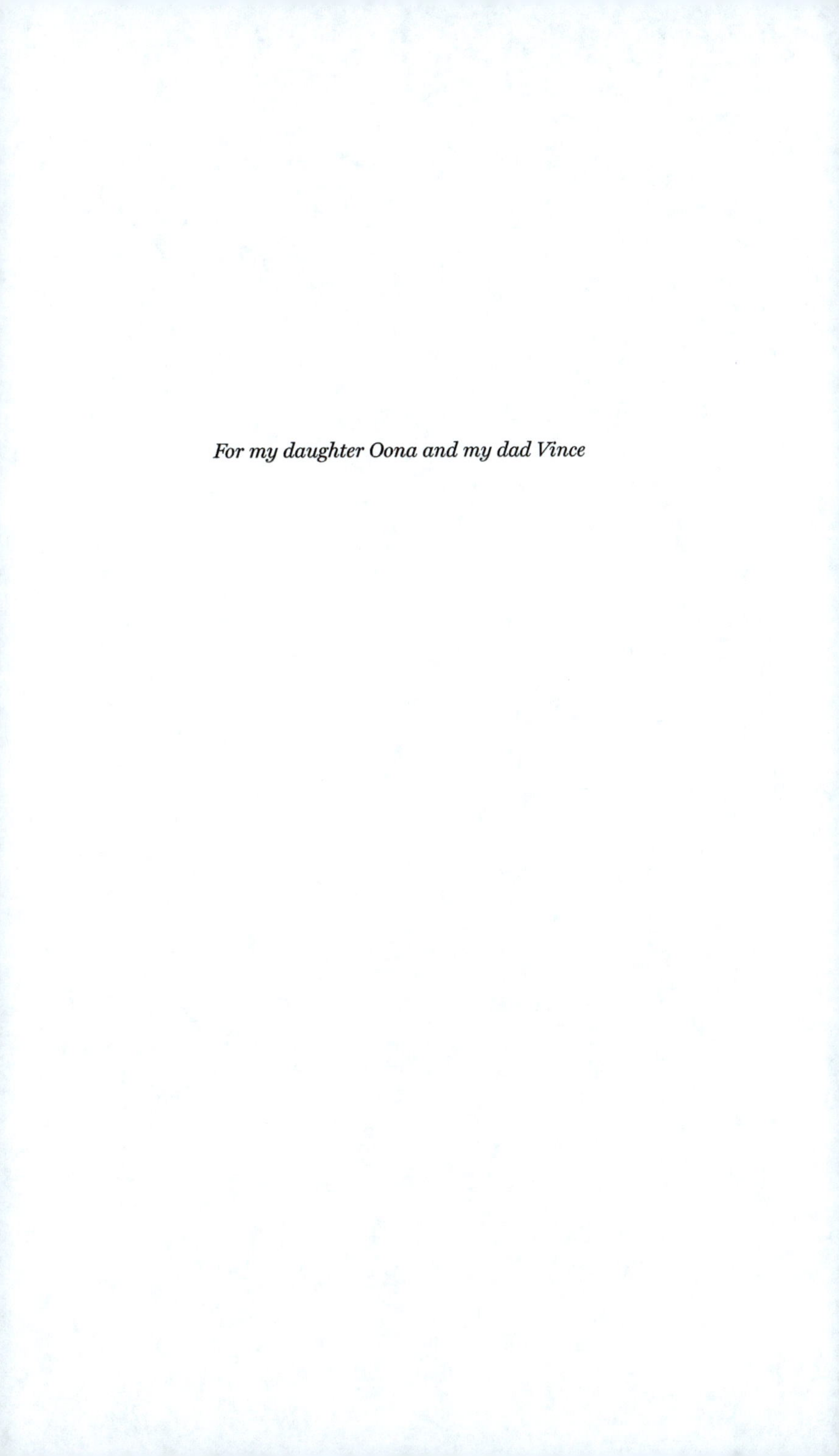

*For my daughter Oona and my dad Vince*

(**MIKE** *enters from offstage.*)

**MIKE**. *(Off audience clapping.)* Thank you guys so much. Thanks for being here. How are ya? Thanks so much.

About a year ago, I'm walking my daughter home from school. She's nine. And my wife and daughter and I live in Brooklyn and they have these smoke shops in my neighborhood with these cutesy names like "Blazy Susan" and "Yes We Can-nabis."

My daughter Oona looks up at the name of one of the shops and goes, "Dad, what's The Good Life?"

I was like, *I don't even know. It's not what I'm doing.*

But I'm thinking I should try to explain what drugs are, so I'm like, "Some people use drugs and they sort of make your brain happy but it's sort of a fake happy and you don't want to get too happy because then you gotta use more drugs to get it as happy as you were the first time and then the ninth or tenth time it's even harder and that's when you're in real trouble. Anyway, Mom and I use them sometimes. Not often. Mostly when we were younger. Not your age. Like...three years older than you are now."

And of course I have to explain drugs to my daughter but no one ever explained them to me. My parents never explained them. The closest was how in sixth grade we had the D.A.R.E. program...which is an acronym that stood for "drug, abuse, resistance, education." Which sorta feels like it was written by someone *on drugs.*

Like, *(Impersonating the D.A.R.E. inventor.)* "It's gotta be four words! And we know what the D is. We're printing the shirts on Monday!"

It was a very shirt-driven campaign. Those shirts are worn to this day ironically by people actively on drugs.

By the way, before the D.A.R.E. program I had never considered using drugs. But after they laid it out I thought I should try these drugs and make an educated decision. Because they made them sound pretty exciting.

They were like, "Kids are gonna come up to you."

I was like, "Keep talking." Kids had never come up to me. This was the most exciting social development of my childhood.

"Kids are gonna come up to you and offer you crank and boomers and angel dust."

I was like, "Angel dust?" I was a sixth grade altar boy. I was like, "I shall try this angel dust and soar to the heavens aside my lord Jesus Christ!"

To this day, I have not been offered crank or boomers or angel dust.

I've never been offered cocaine. I've never even seen cocaine. Sometimes people don't believe me when I say that. I've worked in nightclubs for twenty-three years which are basically cocaine factories and not once has someone thought, *"You know what? We should show it to Mike."*

That's how people see me. I was in Washington Square Park the other day, and a stranger was walking in front of me and someone said to that stranger, "You've got an undercover cop walking behind you."

    *(Looking back twice.)*

And then he looked back at me, and I looked behind me. And there was no one there.

And I said to the stranger, I go, "No..." Which is exactly what an undercover cop would say.

So I've never really used recreational drugs. Even in college when my friends would smoke pot, I was the least fun person to smoke pot with. I was the guy who's like, *"Do you guys hate me? Why does my heart hurt? Is that rickets? Who's at the door? Who's at the door?"* I wasn't a good hang. So I veered away from all that.

I use prescription drugs. I don't want to, but I have to. I have a serious sleepwalking disorder. About twenty years ago I sleepwalked through a second story window of a La Quinta Inn in Walla Walla, Washington, and once you do that once – they *always* bring it up when you go to the doctor. So twenty years ago I was diagnosed with REM Sleep Behavior Disorder, and I've talked about it so much that if you go to med school and you study sleep disorders in the DSM – which is the directory of psychiatric disorders – the example of REM Behavior Disorder...is me.

My dad is a doctor and he wanted me to go to med school. I didn't, but I'm in there. I basically teach.

Two years ago I went to my sleep doctor, I mentioned this to him and he said, "That's not good."

And I go, "What do you mean? We did it!"

He goes, "Well the problem is, I'm not entirely sure that's what you have."

I said, "We're gonna have to write a mass email because there are a lot of people walking around the earth thinking they have Mike Birbiglia disease and Mike Birbiglia might not have it."

Can you imagine if Lou Gehrig was like, "Actually I'm feeling pretty good. I might play baseball again!" People would have been furious. That's right, I just compared myself to Lou Gehrig.

The reason I bring up the sleepwalking disorder is that twenty years ago I get diagnosed with REM Behavior Disorder and they put me on Klonopin. And recently

I went to a new doctor and she's looking at my chart and she goes, "You've been on Klonopin for twenty years?"

And I go, "Yeah."

And she goes, *(Wincing.)* "Alright."

That is not what you wanna hear when you go to the doctor.

She goes, "Are you familiar with the side effects?"

I go, "I don't know."

She goes "Depression, loss of memory, poor motor skills."

I said, "I just thought that was my personality."

It's a strange moment in your life if you realize your personality is *side effects*. So then I'm just self-conscious about my daily activities and it just so happens that my dosage of Klonopin is one and a half milligrams so every night before I go to bed I have to cut a pill precisely in half. You know who shouldn't have a precision task like that? *Someone with poor motor skills.*

Inevitably I break it in half and there's a pile of Klonopin dust on my bathroom sink and I'm so depressed that I'm crying onto the dust and the tears gel with the dust to form a Klonopin sorbet and then *(Explicitly miming licking the surface of a counter.)* I'm licking up what I perceive to be a half of a milligram but definitely isn't half a milligram.

So how do I explain that to my daughter? *"That's the good life! That's what they sell."*

There are so many things I can't explain to my daughter. She's nine years old and it's just getting harder and harder. When they're younger it doesn't matter. They're sort of just an animated bag of rice and you just gotta make sure they stay animated.

And even when they're toddlers the questions are layups.

*"What's that?"*

*"That's an egg!"*

*I'm a genius!*

My wife doesn't know that much either. She's a poet. I'm a comedian. Together we're a sculptor. We don't know a lot. We've read hundreds of books about leaves. We can't explain leaves that well.

This became abundantly clear about a year ago because I get a call from my mom and she said, "Dad has been sick all week and I tried to get him to go to his doctor but he wouldn't go. And then yesterday he fell down in the tub and I called the EMT and they took him to the emergency room and it turned out he had a stroke."

I get off the phone. I'm in my bedroom alone. I go into my closet and I'm just sort of organizing things and I start crying alone.

Then my daughter Oona comes in and she says, "Dad what's wrong?"

I said, "Grandpa Vin had a stroke."

She said, "Dad, what's a stroke?"

That's when I realized...

(*Walking downstage, confiding in audience.*)

I can't fully explain what a stroke is.

I took a swing. I understand the bullet points. It's a brain injury. There's bleeding in your brain.

And then it was a lot of free association after that. I was like, "Your brain is bleeding. I don't know where the blood is. Or was. I think maybe in the vessels. I don't know where they are but now the blood is everywhere. I think. Your body is just filled with blood. Gallons and gallons all over. In a way we're all just sort of bleeding all the time. Maybe ask your mom about that. Or Grandpa. But not this week."

Oona goes, "Is Grandpa Vin gonna be okay?"

I go, "I don't know, I'm gonna go home tonight."

So that night I drive to Providence, Rhode Island, to see my dad at the hospital.

He's in the stroke unit on the seventh floor of Brown University Hospital and when I see him in the gurney he's just this hollowed out version of himself. He can't move half of his body. He can't speak.

The neurologist comes in and she goes, *(Speaking loudly and clearly.)* "Vince – we're gonna do a spinal tap."

My dad just so happens to be a retired neurologist. And from the condition he was in he suggested a specific type of spinal tap.

He said, *(Leaning back so as to impersonate a patient in bed.)* "Guided spinal tap."

Which was impressive. But also, a good example of how controlling my dad is.

I'm watching a half-dead neurologist tell a fully alive neurologist how to do her job. That is next level mansplaining. That's dead-mansplaining. If you don't know the term "mansplaining"... *(To a female audience member in front row.)* It's when a man explains something to a woman that she understands better than he does. I'm not explaining this to you. I'm conveying it. I'm "man-veying."

It was devastating to see my dad like that. Since I was a kid I viewed my dad as larger than life. He was almost like a mythological creature. In a way, I always wanted to be my dad because he knew so much stuff.

My dad was a doctor and in his free time he got his law degree. *(Off audience.)* Yeah. That's how much he didn't want to be a dad. He was like, *"What can I do in these slots of time where I *would* be parenting?"* In fairness we weren't great kids. We always wanted a dad...and he wanted another secondary degree. *(Gesturing in the air to indicate two paths diverging.)* So our goals were at odds.

I never understood my dad's job. I rarely saw that side of him. Sometimes when I was a kid a stranger would come up to me and be like, *(Exaggerated Boston accent.)* *"Yowah dad is a great daw-ctah!"* I'm from *Woostah*, Massachusetts.

I'd be like, "Alright. He's not my doctor."

I didn't know. I mean, who really understands what their parents do for a living?

The other day I was walking Oona home from school and a stranger came up to me and said, "I really like your comedy."

I said, "Aw, thanks."

He says to my daughter, "Your dad is a great comedian."

And she goes, "Alright."

I thought, *"I know what you mean."*

We walked a few blocks and I go, "Oona, what do you think when people say stuff like that?"

She said, "It's a waste of my time."

I thought, *"That's the meanest thing anyone's ever said to me and I know Bill Burr."*

But when I was a kid, I didn't see my dad being a doctor. I mean, every now and then... like I remember one time I was in a soccer game and I was the goalie and I dove headfirst for the ball and I got to it and then a kid on the other team kicked my head with the intensity he had intended for the ball. I don't know the rest of the story. But I have been told...that I hopped up and said, "I'm good!" And they took my word for it and they kept me in the game. About fifteen minutes later, I wander off the field...

> (**MIKE** *walks off stage right, returning from a different, upstage part of stage right.*)

Onto another field...

My teammates go, "Mike, are you okay?"

I said and I quote: "What are we even *doing here*?"

What I remember about that day is that my dad ran onto the field and picked me up and drove me home and he asked me all the questions a neurologist asks when you get a concussion: What's your middle name? What are the classes you take at school? And he was so calm and so focused and I thought, *"My dad is a great doctah."*

The second time I saw that side of my dad was when I was in fifth grade at St. Mary's School where they had a thing called "Science Club" every Friday night. It was kind of like a mafia front for Catholic school. Like, *"We believe Jesus turned water into wine and also...there were dinosaurs."*

Every Friday night a different parent would come to one of the classrooms at St. Mary's and talk about how their job related to science. One week it was gonna be my dad. I was so nervous. I was like, "What's he gonna say? He doesn't know about science."

My dad showed up with his medical tools and he took them out one by one. He took out a three-dimensional model of the brain and explained the hemispheres of the brain. All these kids came up to me afterwards. They were like, *"Yowah dad is wicked smaht. Yowah dad is the smahtest dad."*

I was like, "Yeah. I do have the *smahtest* dad." But how come he didn't explain any of that stuff to me sooner?

That wasn't the version of my dad that I saw. What I would see of my dad is that he would come home from work at about eight o'clock at night and he'd sit in the corner of the living room and read a war novel and scowl. Every now and then he'd fly off the handle about something small.

He'd be like, "WHERE ARE MY GODDAMN KEYS?" I'd be like *(Jogging across the stage.)* "We gotta find those keys!" I spent my whole life looking for those keys. I jumped through a window to get those keys!

My dad would not like that joke.

My mom's solution was to pray. She'd be like "I'm gonna say a prayer to Saint Anthony." Even when I was seven, I was like, "I don't think that's gonna work. We need more concrete tactics to locate the keys."

If you don't know the Christian Saint Anthony, he's the finding stuff guy. Which is sort of a bum deal. Because it's hard to become a saint. You have to perform three miracles. They have to verify the miracles. *(Winking to audience.)* Lotta dark money in that space. Lotta, "Yeah...I saw it."

And then you get canonized if you're lucky. And chances are you find out five minutes before you die. They're like, "Great news! You're gonna be a saint."

You're like, *(Dying.)* "Ahhhhhhh."

They're like "One last thing. You have to find everyone's keys!"

You're like, *(Dying.)* "Nooooooo."

*(Frozen dead.)* And then you're dead.

So I'm with my dad about a year ago in the hospital and it's devastating. If you know someone who's had a stroke, it's the worst thing you could possibly imagine. But I will say – if I'm being completely honest – *it has calmed him down.*

Stay with me. Most of these jokes tonight are for you but a few of them are for me. This is a coping mechanism. I hope it is for you too. This year has been so hard but every once in a while, I think, *"Where was this stroke when I was five?"*

When I was a kid he'd be like, "WHERE ARE MY GODDAMN KEYS?" Now he's like, *(Stilted, as if bedridden.)* "Keys!"

I can't say I don't prefer the latter. It is a little more polite.

*(Walking downstage.)*

Stay with me. It is *my* dad. You can laugh at this. It would be weird if it was your dad, you know what I mean? Like I came out here and am like, "This guy's dad is like…'keys!'"

You'd be like, "Mike has really crossed a line." The most perverse insult comic of all time.

*(Doing an announcer's voice.)* "The Roast of Mike Birbiglia's Audience Members' Ailing Parents!"

So I'm sitting with my dad at the hospital and he can't even really move his face because of the stroke so the only way I can understand his expressions are in his eyes. And the expression in his eyes is fear.

*(Beat.)*

So how do I explain that to my daughter? Pretty sure that's not the good life.

A few days later, I drive home and take my daughter to one of her friend's birthday parties. I go to probably two or three hundred children's birthday parties a year.

It's a huge part of my life. My daughter has six friends. Last year I went to 273 children's birthday parties. The birthday party industrial complex has grown wildly out of control. It's my least favorite part of my life. I don't like it.

I just don't like my daughter's friends. Am I allowed to say that? I love my daughter. I don't like her friends. I don't know if you've spent a lot of time with nine-year-olds you're not related to, but this is an insufferable bunch. I mean when I am with her friends, it makes me *really* not understand pedophilia. *Stay with me.*

*(Tiptoeing across the stage.)*

I'm gonna tiptoe through this minefield of a topic.

You're like, "We weren't with you for the stroke stuff!"

Obviously, I'm evoking the most heinous of crimes, but when I'm with her friends I'm like, *"I don't even get the hook. What's the sell? Who would want to spend any meaningful amount of time with these people? These are our worst and dumbest."* Stay with me – I have examples.

So we're driving to this birthday party and it's me and my wife Jenny, our daughter Oona, and then one of her friends and his dad. And the dads are losers, can we talk about the dads for a sec? Not me! The other dads. They're nothing like me. They're all just dead in the eyes. They've recently developed a stutter. They're always storming into a room like, *"If anyone asks, tell them I tried to find oat milk!"* They're always desperately seeking an alibi for a misdemeanor I'm not familiar with.

So we're heading to this birthday party and we're with one of the dads. His name is Rob. Jenny and I call him "Broccoli Rob."

*(To an audience member.)* Thanks for laughing at that.

Jenny and I think this is hilarious. Broccoli has not laughed once. We have called him this hundreds of times which I think is technically bullying.

Broccoli's son is named Arrow. Which...is a name. By the way, we live in Brooklyn. It's not the only Arrow we know. We know a quiver of Arrows. We know a murder of Beaus.

On the way to the birthday party, we stop at this bakery and this is where nine-year-olds drive me nuts – Arrow says, "Dad, I don't want *wosemary ciabatta*, I want *wegula ciabatta*."

I wanted to say to this kid, "Look, Arrow, life is going to serve you all kinds of ciabatta but if you want to remain true to yourself, hold out for the *wegula*."

So we get the *wegula* ciabatta and we drive from the bakery to this place called Urban Air which, if you're not familiar with this kind of place it's like a birthday party factory. It's a warehouse with trampolines and ice cream and those sticks from American Gladiator that kids can whack each other with. And the moment you enter, you have to sign a stack of forms because they know your child is about to be injured.

They get real specific. It's like, "Your child is about to be stuck under a rusty trampoline."

*(Signing the form.)* "Mike Birbiglia."

"Your child may jump so high her head gets stuck in the rafters."

*(Signing.)* "Mike Birbiglia."

"She may throw up on a rusty trampoline – you will be expected to clean it up with your own mop and bucket available for purchase at the Urban Air store."

*(Signing.)* "Mike Birbiglia."

As you're filling out the forms, the loudspeaker is like,

*(Bearing down on the mic so as to distort the sound.)* "Angelina's birthday in Room 571. Joshua's birthday party in Room 1,310." It's like the seventh circle of hell.

All I want to do is go home. Fortunately, our daughter was injured almost immediately. I say fortunately not because I wish injury upon any child especially not my own, but if it's gonna happen, you want it early. That way you beat the Urban Air rush.

So I drive Jenny and Oona from Urban Air to Urgent Care – which might as well have a shuttle bus. There were a lot of familiar faces over there. I'm not entirely convinced there should be Urgent Care. I'm not sure what they do exactly. I think it was created when someone had a panic attack and was like, *"I need care!"*

And then someone was like, *"When?!"*

And then they're like, *"NOW!"*

Then some well-intentioned person was like "I own this empty building and *(Miming frantically painting the words.)* I can just paint the words 'Urgent Care' on the side and then I'll open my laptop to WebMD.com."

That's all it is, right? Urgent Care is the Urban Air of medicine. Four weeks a year it's a Halloween store. I think that's a red flag.

But we go in and we're frazzled we're like, "Our daughter came down wrong on the trampoline. She hurt her foot."

They were like, "Ahh, sounds like she should see a doctor."

We were like, "No that's why we came here."

They were like "No, we don't know any doctors."

So they sent us to a pediatric orthopedist and the first thing the doctor said was, "We'd like to do an X-ray of her foot."

Oona looks at me and says, "Dad, what's an X-ray?"

*(Beat.)*

I took a swing.

I said, "You get into this machine and then there are these rays that go through your skin and they look around at your bones. *(Miming looking around.)* Then they come back, I think. I don't know how they know how come back. But fingers crossed. Then we hire an artist to draw a picture of your bones based on what the rays have said. Anyway, it's all gonna happen in that room. Mom and I will be out here. We are not allowed anywhere near what's about to happen. It is way too dangerous. There will be technicians in there with you. They will wear bulletproof vests. You will not be wearing one. Don't think too hard about that."

"Take it away, fellas!"

So, she's worried. For good reason – the doctor comes out and says Oona broke one of the bones in her foot and we're gonna put on a cast it.

When your child breaks their foot, it's really like the whole family has broken their collective foot. We brainstormed a lot of foot-free activities like "sitting on couch" or "stewing with anger."

Oona's angry about Arrow because he jumped in front of her on the trampoline. I'm angry about Urban Air. At my lowest point I thought, *"We should sue Urban Air,"* but then I remembered all the paperwork I had signed that explicitly said we would never sue Urban Air. But what the forms don't mention is anything about discussing Urban Air in the context of a comedy show. So, if I were to walk onstage tonight at [the Beacon Theatre] and say, "Urban Air shouldn't be a company" you would know that's a joke.

That's not how I feel about Urban Air. Urban Air is a fantastic company that injures children 365 days a year.

Which is comedic hyperbole. If I walked onstage and said, "Guns don't kill people, Urban Air kills people." We would all know that is a perfect example of satire, your honor.

The Urban Air/Urgent Care situation really hung a lantern on how few things I can explain to my daughter. I can't explain strokes or X-rays or drugs, and increasingly we have to explain sex younger and younger because everyone's devices have access to porn. So now we have to also explain porn. I mean, I can hit the basics, sure. I'm a little hazier on the genres. Even the simple ones like homemade porn have always confounded me. After I have sex all I can think is, "At least no one saw that." I'm never like, "How were we not rolling?! Go again!" *(Aside.)* "It's gonna be forty minutes!"

I certainly never had a sex talk growing up.

When I was about twelve, I had hard nipples...which I'm aware isn't sex.

*(Then.)*

I had hard nipples which is something that happens sometimes during puberty. I say "sometimes" because the first time I built up the courage to share this vulnerable story was with my college roommate and he laughed hysterically for five minutes straight and at the end of the laughter he said to me and I quote: "I think that's just a *you* thing."

So when I was twelve, I had hard nipples and I've always been a hypochondriac so I immediately thought: "cancer." And if you know a hypochondriac, you know that I'm not even exaggerating. I didn't think *maybe* it was cancer. I thought, *"I have cancer. What are the next steps?"* We didn't have urgent care. And I didn't know any doctors, other than my dad.

So one night I walked into the living room and there he was reading his war novel, and I go, "Hey, Dad, I think I might have cancer."

He said, "Why do you think that?"

I said, "I have hard nipples."

He said, "That's not a symptom."

I said, "See for yourself."

And I took off my shirt and he walked over to me, and *(Reaching out as if to mime it.)* he felt my hard, hard nipples...which was nice.

Stay with me. I'm not from a physically affectionate family. We don't say I love you. We don't hug. So when my dad caressed my hard, hard nipples I thought, *"It's not 'I love you' but I'll take it."*

Then my father, Dr. Vince Birbiglia, gave me the briefest medical diagnosis I have received to this very day. He goes, "Nope."

That was the end of the conversation. That was the closest to a sex talk that I would receive for the rest of my life.

We weren't a physically affectionate family. I mean every now and then... When I was five years old, I was dangerously dehydrated. It's called being "hypotonic." My mom drove me to the emergency room and they wouldn't put an IV in me because we hadn't filled out the right insurance form. So she's manically filling out these insurance forms. My dad shows up and he shouts, *(Yelling.)* "GIVE THAT GODDAMN KID AN IV!"

And they did it immediately. Which was a weird affirmation of my dad's dysfunctional personality.

I don't even remember that part of it. But what I do remember is I was admitted into the hospital for four days and one day my dad came in – it was just me and him – and he brought me a Curious George doll. I kept it through my entire childhood.

> *(Slowly, reaching out to the air to mime rubbing a shoulder.)*

And he rubbed my shoulder for about fifteen minutes. It was the slightest gesture but I remember it to this day.

Jenny and I are the opposite with our daughter. We are too much. Whatever too much is, we're gonna find out when she's an adult. We say I love you. We hug her. We squeeze her.

A few years ago we went to her ballet recital and we're in the audience just crying and crying. 'Cause she doesn't have it. I mean, we're in the arts. We have a sense for these things. There are a lot of early indicators.

No. We're crying because we've spent thousands of dollars on lessons and hundreds of hours going to rehearsal and she's not going pro.

No, we're crying for the right reasons. After the recital I run up to her and I'm squeezing her and I say, "Oona! You were so fantastic."

And she said, "Dad, you would say I was fantastic even if I wasn't fantastic."

And I had to say "That is so true. You are so much better at logic than you are at ballet."

I left out that last snippet. I'm gonna save that until she's fifteen and she tells me I'm garbage and I'll say, "I had some candid thoughts about you as well when you were seven that I withheld out of respect but I did share with a group of strangers at [the Beacon Theatre in New York City]."

We do withhold sometimes.

I mean, for example, I experience anger, but I keep it in. Because when I was a kid and my dad would get angry, I remember thinking, *"I am never gonna do that."*

Because kids don't know a lot but they absorb everything. If you're selfish, your kids know you're selfish. If you're kind, they know you're kind.

A few months ago, Oona noticed that when I woke up, Jenny had made me pancake. You heard that correctly... it was just one. She made me "pancake."

I said, "Thank you for pancake."

And it really was thoughtful because she's deeply familiar with my health profile so she knows the right amount of pancakes for me to eat is "pancake."

So I wanted to do something nice for her because my love language is keeping score. *(Addressing an audience member who is clapping.)* If you're clapping yours is too. And if you're not clapping yours is too, but you're losing. You just didn't know there was a game going on.

Last year Jenny said to me, "Sometimes I feel like you're keeping score," and I was like, "Right. I'm not being coy about it. What do you think the white board is for in the kitchen?"

I keep score and I wish I were more subtle about it. Jenny describes me as, "The narrator of our marriage who nobody asked for."

I'll be scrubbing dishes in the sink and I'll be like, "So I'm doing the dishes. Then I'm gonna grab ice cream because your parents are coming over and then I'm gonna take the hair out of the drain in the shower."

She'll be like, "You don't have to say all that. You could just do it. And then it'll be done. And we don't have to talk about. I do a lot of stuff too. I don't talk about it. I just do it. And then it's done."

I'm like, "We're gonna give you five points for that one on the whiteboard." *(Miming drawing on the white board.)* "You're still down by three, it doesn't matter."

I'm not proud of keeping score. I don't know if I learned it from my parents. I mean, I just don't know how to be married. No one taught me this. I'm just winging it every day. My marriage doesn't look anything like my parents' marriage. My parents argued all the time when I was a kid.

Jenny and I don't argue in the same way because Jenny is an introvert. Arguing with an introvert is just reading into the silences and deciding which of the silences you want to have words.

The other day Jenny and I were walking to pick up our daughter at school and she seemed quiet, and I go, "What's wrong?"

And she goes "Nothing."

But it wasn't nothing. It was one of those forks in the road where I'm like, *"Wait. Do I probe or do I let it lie?"*

> *(Beat, walking downstage.)*

*(Directly into the microphone.)* Does anyone know?

> **(MIKE** *looks out into the audience to seek their counsel.)*

Who's been married the longest? Shout out how many years you've been married if you think you're married the longest.

*(Responding to a specific audience member.)* How long have you been married? What are your names?

> *(NOTE: Audience responses vary here. In the following example the couple's names are Linda and Bill and they have been together for forty-nine years. Take improvisational*

*liberties based on the subsequent audience interaction.)*

*(Then.)*

[So Bill and Linda have been married forty-nine years.] My parents have been married sixty years. That is too long. There should be term limits. One time in my twenties I said to my mom this thing that I felt like I wanted to say for years. I said, "Mom, I want you to know, if you ever wanted to divorce Dad, we would understand."

And I thought she was gonna be like, *(Miming a fist bump.)* "Thanks."

But I'll never forget what she said. She said, "Michael, you cannot understand someone else's marriage."

Which is all to say, [Linda]…if you ever wanted to get divorced I would be okay with it.

*(Then.)*

No, the reason I ask is that you've been married a long time. If you're in this situation, [Linda]. Where you say to [Bill], "What are you thinking about?" and he says, "Nothing." Would you probe or let it lie?

*(Let audience respond.)*

[Is Bill here? Bill, would you probe or let it lie?] *(If Bill isn't present.)* [If Bill were here, would he say probe or let it lie?]

*(All different improvs follow depending on the audience participation. Listen carefully and respond specifically. "And that is why the marriage has lasted forty-nine years," etc.)*

Anyway, the point is: I probed. I generally think it's better to know more than less.

I said to Jenny, "What are you thinking about?"

She said, "Nothing." She doubled down on it.

So I threw an off-speed pitch. I said, "Where did you come from just now?"

She said, "I was at home watching the news and I got sad about the war."

I said, "Do you think it's my fault?"

I was raised Catholic so I'm open to the idea that anything could be my fault. I think it's entirely possible that I masturbated so much that it caused a war in the Middle East. Maybe I'm a dreamer but I'm pretty sure that's what that song is about.

My dad would not like that joke. He wouldn't like a lot of my jokes. He particularly doesn't like it when they're crude. Or also personal. Like for example, I don't think he would have loved the five-minute section on hard nipples.

And he doesn't like political jokes. As a matter of fact, when I was in my twenties, I was doing this political joke and it sparked a discussion between me and him about politics and it was tense. I was visiting him and we went on a walk on this wooded path near his house. The farther we walked, the more tense it got. At a certain point, he was just saying mean-spirited things about me, and then I started to say mean-spirited things about him.

When I got back to my car to drive home I said, "Bye, Dad."

He didn't say goodbye. He goes, "Well...you've gone another way."

That was it. I'm driving home and I felt so adrift. I thought my whole life I sort of wanted to be my dad but at a certain point I decided I wanted him to be me.

I never had that with my mom. We've always been close since I was a kid because she's very religious and I was too because kids love magic.

I always wanted to be a priest because they got so many laughs on such little material. They'd be like, "Matthew, Mark, Luke, and *John Boy!*"

People would be like, "Father Patrick's hilarious!"

I'd be like, "He's not hilarious. There are no punchlines. It's all set-ups." I was just like, *"Get me up there. Put me on the mic. Sign me up for some open altars."* I would kill... I would crucify.

They didn't let me become a priest because I was ten so I became an altar boy and the answer is no I wasn't. I think it's because they knew I was a talker. I have that look about me and I think they thought, *"If he's this bad at lighting candles, he's not gonna be great at blowing them out."*

*(Off audience.)* No I know, for some people, that's too much. But I think what the priests did was too much. I don't think the jokes about it are nearly as bad. I don't think we should let it lie.

It's hard to describe to my friends how religious my upbringing was. Sometimes it comes up. Like, the other day I was in an Uber with Jenny, and this hymn from childhood just flew into my head.

It was this hymn that goes:

> (**MIKE** *sings a line from a well-known Catholic hymn.*[*])

All of those lyrics went straight into my head in an Uber to CVS. You cannot be cured of this religion. It is

---

*A license to produce *The Good Life* does not include a performance license for any third-party or copyrighted music. Licensees should create an original composition or use music in the public domain. For further information, please see the Music and Third-Party Materials Use Note on page iii.

the forever chemicals of religions.

So I look over at Jenny in the Uber. I go, "This hymn just came into my head."

And then I sang it to her, like I sang it to you. But she didn't laugh. She was just stone faced.

But I was like, "No, but it's funny right?!" And then I just sang it louder.

She still had a very serious face.

And then she texted me from three inches away from me. I was like, *"Uh oh."*

I look at my phone and it's a text from Jenny that says: *The Uber driver has rosary beads hanging on his rear view mirror.*

I'm an improvisor so I said, "The reason I'm bringing up that hymn is because it's very meaningful to me and I would like to teach it to you. So repeat after me:"

*(He starts singing the hymn again.)*

I actually had my own rosary beads as a kid. My grandmother gave them to me for my first communion. If you don't know what rosary beads are, they're like an abacus for Catholic people that counts your prayers. If you don't know what an abacus is, it's like a calculator. A Catholic calculator.

Every night before bed I'd take out my rosary beads and pray. I would do Hail Marys and Our Fathers and Glory Bes. My whole childhood, my consciousness was me and God. And then at a certain point, it was just me.

In May of last year, I'm visiting my dad in the hospital and my mom is praying. I'm not praying but I'm sort of backup dancing, you know what I mean? (**MIKE** *circles around the stage in a makeshift backup dancing performance, singing nonsensically as he moves.)* I'm "yes and-ing" the situation.

My mom is praying because my dad has gotten worse. In addition to not being able to move, he has a blockage in his stomach and it got so bad his stomach was distended by about five inches and they put an NG tube down his throat to suck out the gas and the liquid.

He's in agony. He says to me, "Michael, I'm dying."

And I said, "Dad I don't think you're dying."

*(Beat.)*

But I didn't know.

The next morning I get a call from the comedian Jim Gaffigan. I've known Jim for years but he had a slightly different tone.

He says, *(Squinting.)* "Hey um, so the Pope – Pope Francis – wants to meet some comedians at the Vatican and apparently you're on the list and I'm on the list and I don't know… I'm gonna go."

I said, "Does the Pope know that if he invites comedians, we'll probably talk about it onstage?"

Jim goes, "He's gotta know… but maybe go easy on the molestation stuff."

I thought, *I will when they do. You first, Catholic Church."*

*(If the audience is cheering.)* Don't clap, because then it becomes a rally.

My first inclination was to say no because for years my parents have encouraged me to take Oona to church and we haven't gone, not because of anything anti-religious, if anywhere had that kind of track record… I mean if there were a Whole Foods that had a series of molestations, we wouldn't shop there anymore. Even if they were like, "It only happens sometimes."

I'd be like, "I think that's my number. I think 'sometimes' is my limit."

But then I'm with my dad at the hospital and I said, "I got invited to meet the Pope." And he lit up like Grandpa Joe in *Charlie and the Chocolate Factory*. *(Lighting up.)* And that's when I realized I was going to Vatican City to meet the Pope.

In June I get plane tickets for me and Jenny and Oona. We to fly to Rome. We're walking around the Vatican. I found it surprisingly emotional. It's a stunning place of course and then I'm explaining to Oona, "This is the religion I was raised in. Grandma MJ believes in a lot of this stuff. I believe in some of it. And a lot of this artwork was stolen. You shouldn't steal artwork, but if you do…don't give it back. That's the lesson of the Vatican. If you steal, steal big and don't give it back."

Then Oona asks me a question that really took me by surprise. She says, "Dad, who is Jesus?"

(**MIKE** *puts his head in his hands.*)

I thought, *"This is a major oversight in my education of my daughter."* Because she knows the Greek gods and the Roman gods and the Norse gods and the Egyptian gods. Somehow I have entirely glossed over Jesus.

So I'm trying to do a crash course. I'm like, "He's this guy from 2,000 years ago and some people think he was the son of God but also God and he had this cult – it was like a well-meaning cult."

Which, by the way, that's not even controversial. If Jesus were here onstage with me here at [the Beacon Theatre] he'd be like "Yeah it was a cult. There were twelve of us. Seventy tops!"

Jesus would be baffled by what happened to Christianity. He'd be like, "This isn't what I intended at all. I'm more like a cross between David Blaine and a food bank."

By the way, no offense to cults.

Some offense to cults.

I don't support cults, but Jenny and I always get into the documentaries about them.

The first episode always feels promising. It's all about carpooling and shared meals. We're like, "This could work." We're looking it up on Google Maps like, *"Where is this place?"*

Second episode goes dark. It's like, "Then we had to have sex with Leader."

I'm always like: how often? There's a hundred of you. How often are you in the rotation? Once a month? Once every three months?

You know how many things I do every three months that are worse than sex with Leader? Put it on the calendar! That's the key to any great marriage. You gotta get it in the calendar. Sometimes I'll have sex with Leader. Sometimes Jenny will have sex with Leader. Sometimes I'll have sex with Jenny and call her "Leader." Count it!

By the way I should clarify my tone when discussing cults. I recently received an email from an audience member who wrote, "We really enjoyed the show but I want you to know that if you *did* join a cult, you should know that Jenny would have to have sex with leader more often than you would have to have sex with leader."

And this really spun me out. I thought I must not be conveying my humor properly if this person leaves the show thinking that A. I might join a cult. And B. if I joined a cult, I don't know that Jenny would have to have sex with Leader more often than I would have to have sex with Leader.

So I want to take this moment in the show to point out...some of these are jokes.

The point is I'm in Rome with my family. It's interesting because everywhere you go in Rome there are paintings of Jesus and statues of Jesus to the point where I said to the tour guide, *"Was he here?* I went to Catholic school and I know he wasn't, but you guys kinda make it feel like he was."

In some ways Rome is the original culprit of cultural appropriation. Because Jesus never got the fun parts of Rome. *(Speaking in an exaggerated Italian accent.)* He didn't get *the pizza* and *the pasta* and he didn't get to say *"mamma mia!"* with his buddies. All Jesus knows about Rome is the Romans showed up at his cult in Jerusalem and they're like, "We love what you're doing, It's a great story. A classic rags to rags. But we think it would be more compelling if the protagonist died." And then they murdered him.

*(Off audience.)* I know. It wasn't me.

But the even more perverse side of it is that they killed him and then they sold paintings of themselves murdering him to take over half the world. That's like if the Wilkes Booth family sold Lincoln Logs.

So I explain this to the Pope and he thinks it's hilarious. But he doesn't speak English, so who's to say?

No, the truth is that the comedians didn't perform for the Pope. Which I felt like was a missed opportunity because it was people like Chris Rock and Stephen Colbert and Whoopie Goldberg and David Sedaris. And me.

Which, by the way, I get that I was at the bottom of that list. I got the call in May and the trip was in June. I'm pretty sure there was an April list.

They got some "no"s and then the Pope was googling "comedian" on his Dell laptop and his last name is "Bergoglio" and my last name is "Birbiglia" and I think he was like, *(Speaking in an exaggerated Italian accent.)* *"He's a Birbiglia and I'mma Bergoglio. It's-a my long-a-lost-a cousin!"*

He doesn't talk like that. He's not even Italian. He's from Buenos Aires but I'm not sure the comedy community cleared that accent yet, so until then... *Mamma mia! I'mma the Pope-a! We make a pizza pie outta the Eucharist.*

We didn't perform any jokes for the Pope. The Pope spoke to us, *about comedy.* Which is a perfect example of how power corrupts. I don't know how you get to a point of thinking you're so good at being a priest that you're like, "I'm gonna invite Chris Rock over to my house and tell him *my* take on comedy."

That's like if I showed up at NASA and said, "I got some thoughts about rockets. I think it's important that we build them and then fly them but never on the outside like in cartoons. And that concludes my presentation on rockets. Now everyone kiss my wedding ring."

Everyone's like, *"Ew, it's sweaty."*

The Pope spoke to us about comedy. And if you don't know Pope Francis, he's a pretty good pope, but only compared to other popes. If you met him at a party you'd be like, *"This fucking guy?"* But compared to other popes, he's amazing.

He invited us into what's called the "The Apostolic Palace" and he gave a speech about humor. It was about forty minutes long, but I jotted down my favorite parts.

> (**MIKE** *takes out the translation from his pocket.*)

It was in Italian but they gave us a translation.

He said:

*(Reading from paper.)*

*Dear friends – in the midst of so much gloomy news, immersed as we are in many social and personal emergencies, you have the power to spread smiles. You are among the few that have the ability to speak to all types of different people from different generations and cultural backgrounds.*

It was sweet. Good, friendly Pope stuff.

Then he said:

*According to the Bible...*

This is where he loses me a little bit.

*At the beginning of the world, while everything was being created, divine wisdom practiced your form of art for the benefit of none other than God himself, the first spectator of history.*

Which I have to say has always been one of the more unnerving aspects of Catholicism – this idea that God is the spectator of everything. They taught us that at St. Mary's grade school because they said, "God is watching you at all times." I took that literally. I was seven and I just assumed it was some guy tailing me in a Chevy Malibu. Like, "What's Mike Birbiglia up to? Oh, he's hiding porn in the forest? I'm gonna make sure he doesn't have a girlfriend 'til he's twenty." That prophecy came true so maybe there is a God.

That imagery really stuck with me through my childhood. When I was fifteen, I started masturbating, and I remember thinking, "I guess he's watching me do that too." So I would sort of cheat to the camera because I wanted to think if he happened to glance at the monitor at that moment, he would be like, "I've seen a lot of fifteen-year-olds masturbate, but this kid's good! I think he might go pro." And I have. Which is a happy ending. Not technically. Alright, then the Pope said:

*I am reminded of the story in the book of Genesis when God promised Abraham that within a year he would have a son. He and his wife Sarah were old and childless.*

She was twenty-three.

*Sarah conceived and bore a son in her old age.*

Twenty-four.

*Then Sarah said, "God has made laughter for me." That is why they named their son Isaac, which means, "he laughs."*

Then finally he said:

*Remember this: when you manage to draw smiles from the lips of even one spectator, you also make God smile.*

I thought that was nice.

And then he gave us rosary beads that he had blessed in a little green satchel.

I brought them home to my parents in July. It was my dad's eighty-fourth birthday. It was me, my mom, my brother Joe, my sister Gina, my sister Patti, and all of our kids – my dad's six grandkids. We're all around my dad in his little condo celebrating this man's unlikely eighty-fourth birthday.

I gave him the rosary beads blessed by the Pope and he lit up. Then my mom said to me, "You were called by God."

*(Walking downstage, confiding in audience.)*

I want you to know...I don't think I was called by God. What I wanted to say was, "No. I was called by Jim Gaffigan." Who was called by Stephen Colbert – who may have been called by God.

But when your parents have had a year like my mine have had, you find yourself saying things like "Yes, I was called by God."

We had a cake for my dad and then everyone headed home and I'm just standing there with my dad, and he's lying in his bed. He's able to talk but doesn't remember anything that happened the past year. So I just ask him questions about things that happened a long time ago.

He was born in 1940, in Bushwick, Brooklyn. I said, "When you were growing up was your family coming back from World War II?"

He goes, "Yes, my Uncle Charlie. My Uncle Tony. My Uncle Joe. They all came back with wild stories about how they were nearly killed."

I said, "Did you get drafted for Vietnam?"

He said, "Yes, I was in the draft but they decided to send me as a doctor to a base in Texas so we lived there for three years. And we met some of our closest friends for our whole lives."

And I said, "What was your address when you were a kid growing up in Brooklyn?"

He tells me his address and I show him on my phone that it's four miles from his childhood home to his granddaughter Oona's childhood home. I showed it to him.

I thought, *"How come my dad never told me any of this stuff sooner?"*

Then I thought, *"How come I hadn't asked?"*

My dad at this point is tired and can't really speak anymore but I want to connect with him because when your dad is eighty-four, you don't know how many more times you'll get to see him again. So I reach over and I start rubbing his shoulder.

> (**MIKE** *begins acting out rubbing his father's shoulder.*)

I could tell from his eyes he enjoyed it. His cheeks crested up a little. I rubbed his arm for about fifteen minutes and I felt as close to my dad as I did when he brought me the Curious George doll in the hospital, and when I was twelve and he caressed my hard, hard nipples.

The next day I drive Jenny and Oona home to Brooklyn.

A few days later I'm walking Oona home from school and I think to myself, *"That's all I can really teach my daughter. We will never know everything. We will all often be wrong, no matter how hard we probe. And it's possible small acts of kindness are all we have. And maybe...that's the good life."*

*(Fade to black, end of show.)*